NUTRITION FOR ATHLETES

Contents

Since consuming more of these foods is often simpler than following an avoidance diet, you may find it useful to concentrate on these items. Of all, your body differs from everyone else's, so it's possible that certain meals may help you perform faster than others.

Bananas are an excellent source of sustained energy without the chance of a sugar crash since they are low in calories and sugar content. Bananas have a high fiber level, which can help you feel fuller for longer and promote post-workout recovery. The 422 mg of potassium included in an average banana can assist your body manage fluid balance, lowering your risk of cramps and spasms. Because potassium is lost via perspiration during exercising, athletes should consume enough potassium-rich foods afterward to maintain healthy levels.

If you don't have an egg allergy or intolerance, eggs are a fantastic source of protein, healthy fats, calcium, vitamin B, and other nutrients. Several natural energy sources, including vitamins B1, B2, B6, and B12, are found in eggs, which may assist improve your performance. Eggs contain a lot of choline, which helps to increase endurance and prevents weariness. Eggs include magnesium, which may aid in healing, and zinc, which is good for gaining lean muscle mass.

Food energy

Athletes have higher energy requirements than the normal individual. Male and female athletes often require more than 2,400–3,000 kcal and 2,200–2,700 kcal per day, respectively, particularly those who are still developing. The macronutrient (carbohydrate, protein, and fat) composition of a meal determines how much energy it contains

Tips to excel with proper sports nutrition

Plan to consume a range of fruits and vegetables each day. At least five servings per day should be consumed, with a variety of fruit and vegetable colours. The size of a serving is around that of a baseball. The nutrients and energy needed for exercise and recuperation are abundant in fruits and vegetables. Additionally, these meals will aid in your fight against diseases like the flu and the common cold.

Improve endurance with beet juice

ImpBeets are rich in the carbs essential for long-lasting energy as well as several anti-inflammatory and antioxidant elements. Beets' strong nitrate content may also aid in blood vessel dilation. Both the blood pressure and the quantity of oxygen given to the cells may be lowered as a result.

According to a research cited by the American Heart AssociationTrusted Source, drinking one cup of beet juice each day may help decrease blood pressure and improve blood flow.

build stamina with beet juice

ACHIEVING DESIRED WEIGHTS FOR COMPETITIVE PURPOSES

If you want to change your body weight to perform better, you must do it carefully or it can have the opposite effect. Negative health impacts might result from maintaining a body weight that is too low, decreasing weight too rapidly, or preventing weight increase in an unnatural manner. Setting realistic body weight goals is crucial.

Working with a qualified dietician is recommended for young athletes who are attempting to reduce weight. Individual diet experimentation might result in unhealthy eating patterns and an insufficient or excessive intake of certain nutrients.

To discuss a diet that is appropriate for your sport, age, sex, and quantity of training, speak with a health care expert.

PROTEIN

Protein is necessary for bodily tissue repair and muscular development. The body can also utilise protein as an energy source, but only when glucose reserves have been depleted.

But it's also untrue that eating a lot of protein can help you gain muscle.

Muscle can only be changed through exercise and strength training.

Only a little amount of additional protein is required by athletes, including bodybuilders, to promote muscle development. By consuming more total calories, athletes may easily fulfil this increased need (eating more food).

The average American already consumes about twice as much protein as they need for muscular growth. The diet contains too much protein:

Will be kept as additional body fat may raise the risk of being dehydrated (not getting enough fluids in the body), which can cause calcium loss.
may make the kidneys work harder
The most significant source of energy during exercise is carbs, which are often insufficient for those who place a high priority on consuming more protein.

It is not advised to use amino acid supplements or consume a lot of protein.

Eat Extra for Excellence

The great news about food for games is that you don't need a particular diet or supplements to perform at your best. It all comes down to incorporating the proper nutrients in the proper quantities into your training regimen.

Compared to their less active classmates, teen athletes have distinct nutritional demands. Athletes work out more, thus they need more calories to fuel their development as well as their athletic performance.

Athletes and Dieting

Teen athletes need more nourishment, therefore dieting is often not a good option. In weight-focused sports like wrestling, swimming, dancing, or gymnastics, athletes may experience pressure to slim down. However, severely reducing calories may impair development and increase the risk of bones and other injuries.

If a coach, fitness instructor, or teammate advises you to diet, speak with your doctor first or seek out a dietician who focuses on young athletes. If a medical expert you trust says dieting is safe, they may collaborate with you to develop a healthy eating strategy.

Eat a Variety of Foods

Eating wholesome, nutritious meals and snacks can help you acquire the nutrition your body needs to fuel your game for the long haul. You may get advice on what sorts of foods and beverages to include in your diet from the MyPlate food pyramid.

essential minerals and vitamins
Teen athletes require a range of nutrients from their diets in addition to the recommended daily intake of calories in order to maintain their performance levels. Minerals and vitamins are among them. Iron and calcium are two essential elements for athletes:

Athletes rely on their strong bones, which calcium helps to develop. Dairy products including low-fat milk, yoghurt, and cheese include calcium, which is essential for preventing stress fractures.
Apples
It could be true that "one apple a day keeps the doctor away" after all! Apples are rich in pectin, a fibre, and slow-release carbohydrates,

which aid to strengthen the heart and control blood sugar levels in the body. The amphoteric activity of pectin. Depending on what the body requires, apples may help with both diarrhoea and constipation. Apples are also rich in quercetin, which has anti-inflammatory and anticancer properties.

Blackberries

These little health dynamos are packed with antioxidants that shield us from heart conditions. Blackberries combat free-radical damage in the body and handle a number of contemporary disorders including hypertension, diabetes, cancer, eyesight loss, impaired liver function, and deteriorating mental abilities because of their high antioxidant content. Magnesium, zinc, iron, and calcium are abundant in them. Their high vitamin E concentration keeps skin healthy and protects the heart.

Fruit and Vegetables for Improved Exercise Performance

Many individuals who are dedicated to sports, fitness, and strength training sometimes fail to see the significance of consuming a range of fruits and vegetables. These foods may affect stamina, performance, and endurance. While many people are aware of the significance of protein, carbs, and fat, they tend to overlook the significance of the micronutrients included in fruits and vegetables.

In order to maintain health and maximise exercise performance, energy generation, and tissue healing during times of exercise training, fruits and vegetables' micronutrient content is crucial. In order to sustain daily exercise and recuperation, a person must eat a diet high in fruits and vegetables since certain nutrients the body cannot synthesise.

An inadequate diet of fruits and vegetables may cause tiredness, muscular injury, weakness, and immune system impairment, all of which can have a negative impact on training and recuperation for competitions or overall sports performance and fitness.

Athletes and those who engage in intense exercise may also be at higher risk for disease and infection. Due to a greater demand for antioxidants, individuals must consume more of these essential nutrients, which they may do by eating more fruits and vegetables. Juicing is a fantastic approach to meet that additional need. A regular diet with five to seven servings of fruits and vegetables was recommended as the most helpful treatment in a research that examined the anti-oxidants in exercise.

What An Athlete Needs From Their Food

In order to maintain high levels of dietary energy, athletes need to consume more calories than the normal person.

Carbohydrates are the main source of dietary energy for high-intensity exercises. Dietary protein aids in muscle development and repair, whereas dietary fat aids in the absorption of fat-soluble vitamins, serves as a backup energy source, and maintains balanced hormone levels.

Fat is the body's primary energy source. Fat is the body's primary energy source while it is at rest. When a person starts doing high-intensity exercise, their body starts using carbs as their primary source of energy for their muscles and brain.

Let's examine the key dietary categories for athletes.

Unhealthy Eating Habits to Avoid

Since food plays such a significant role in an athlete's physique, bad eating habits may make it challenging to perform at your best. Important nutrients including potassium, fibre, vitamin D, and calcium are often insufficient in the diets of many individuals. Be careful to refrain from the following bad habits:

Meal skipping: Finding time to eat breakfast before leaving the house might be challenging at times, but missing meals can hurt your athletic performance, particularly if you aren't getting the necessary amount of calories.

Making selections about snacks may be difficult, particularly when processed, sugary foods are readily available. When picking snacks, look for entire meals that have healthful nutrients. Try to plan your snacks for the day in advance or stock your cupboard with better selections.

Using diets or other weight-loss techniques: A lot of fad diets and weight-loss methods might hurt rather than improve your performance, so beware of them. Do you envision yourself following this diet at this time next year? The likelihood is that the strategy is not ideal for you if the response is no.

Timing and regularity of meals: Setting up a nutritious eating routine will make it easier to satisfy your nutritional needs without having to put too much thought into it. Additionally, your body will adapt to the timetable. A 3- to 5-hour interval between meals is suggested as an eating regimen. This enables optimal levels of satiety, blood sugar regulation, and correct digestion.

Unbalanced nutrition: Consuming too much of one nutrient might have a negative impact on function. For continuing muscle growth and recuperation, protein and carbohydrates in particular are highly helpful nutrients, therefore you must consume enough of each daily.

unhealthy food choices One thing to keep in mind when making a meal plan for an athlete is that the foods you choose do matter. While not all of the food you consume has to be organic and nutritious, a balanced plate is essential for increasing your muscle mass and endurance.

EGGS

The finest protein for athletes may be found in eggs. Eggs are a good source of lecithin minerals including zinc, iron, and copper as well as vitamins like A, B2, B6, D, E, and K. In addition, eggs include choline and betaine, both of which may support a heart-healthy lifestyle for athletes. Eggs from chickens, quail, and ducks are among the most often used types. For the benefit of athletes, eggs from free-range or organically kept hens are higher quality and more enriched.

GRAINS

Athletes must consume whole grains high in fibre. This kind of meal may considerably lower cholesterol levels and lower the dangers of diabetes, obesity, and stroke. A few whole grains also include important amino acids and other minerals including calcium, potassium, and iron. Amaranth, teff, oats, brown rice, barley, whole wheat, sorghum, maize, and rye are some examples of grains that fit into this group.

HEALTHY FATS

All fats are not harmful. For instance, unsaturated fats assist decrease dangerous cholesterol levels, which lessens the damaging impact on health. Additionally, the body needs these good fats for proper operation. As a result, athletes should consume meals that contain this crucial component. Avocado oil, salmon fish oil, olive oil, and nut oils are a few examples of these good fats.

The diet of an athlete has a big impact on how well they perform. However, finding and planning diets that fit individual nutritional demands takes a lot of work. Athletes have the chance to save time by using Fit Five to organise their dietary requirements. Athletes may easily acquire nutritious meals thanks to the many meal packs and delivery options. Contact the Fit Five staff right now to learn more about our meal programmes.

WATER, VITAMINS, AND MINERALS

Vegetables have several benefits for athletes, but their major benefit is that they help athletes stay hydrated, which is one of the factors that might affect performance. It spreads to the cells after digestion since they are inherently quite rich in water. Our food intake accounts for around 40% of our water consumption. Fruits and vegetables account for a significant portion of this consumption.

The vitamin and antioxidant content of veggies is another benefit they provide. In addition to providing the nutrients needed for maintaining muscle tone, vegetables like spinach, bell peppers, cabbage, tomatoes, and others also help to reverse any harm caused by free radicals produced during stressful situations or vigorous exercise.

Vegetables are an excellent source of nutrients and trace elements that support neuromuscular transmission (the delivery of commands to the muscles) and aid in the recovery process after exertion.

COMPLEX CARBOHYDRATES AND THE ATHLETE

Similar to pasta and rice, dry legumes (beans, lentils, chickpeas, etc.) supply complex carbohydrates that provide energy (glucose) to working muscles. As a result, dry legumes, like pasta and rice, are crucial that they have no health advantages. Artificial sweeteners deceive the body into believing you're ingesting genuine food, and because they're almost 100 times sweeter than the actual thing, your body begins to produce insulin as a result (the fat storage hormone). The genuine material is best to consume in modenutrients to promote physical exertion. Even better, you may mix both (starch +

dry legume) to increase calorie intake, provide a well-balanced supply of plant-based protein, and enhance digestion.

Diet Soda

Each meal is seen by athletes as a chance to refuel: How much protein can I pack into this meal? How can I include more healthy fats? It is the force behind performance. Artificial sweeteners and other non-nutritional foods have no place in their diet. A Purdue University research found that artificially sweetened items like a can of diet Coke might greatly raise your risk for health issues and weight gain in addition to the fact that they have no health advantages. Artificial sweeteners deceive the body into believing you're ingesting genuine food, and because they're almost 100 times sweeter than the actual thing, your body begins to produce insulin as a result (the fat storage hormone). The genuine material is best to consume in moderation.

What are the Worst Foods to Eat Pre-Competition?

Foods that take longer to digest upset the stomach when eaten. Blood from the digestive tract is diverted by the body to boost athletic performance. This denotes concerns with digestion such as poor digestion, stomach distress, and more. This result will result from eating too much protein, fat, and fibre.

High fat foods include fried foods, greasy pizza, fatty meat cuts, ice cream, cake, cookies, and chips, among other things.

High fibre foods include beans, cruciferous vegetables like broccoli, cauliflower, and Brussels sprouts, certain fruits with skin, chia seeds, flax seeds, and others.

High protein — A little amount of protein with pre-event meals and snacks might be beneficial, but too much protein can cause problems. Avoiding the protein supplement at this time could be the wisest course of action.

Non-nutritive sweeteners: Since the body cannot efficiently break down these sweet additions, they do not provide useful energy. While many people prefer the lack of calories, this property implies an athlete does not get the necessary energy and may face GI discomfort like bloating or diarrhoea since these components are not properly digested.
Stevia, artificial sweeteners, and sugar alcohols are examples of non-nutritive sweeteners. Athletes should be wary of meals and drinks labelled as "light" or "sugar-free," since these items often include artificial sweeteners.

Spicy foods: These foods might cause digestive problems and induce heartburn. Athletes should use care while consuming these items.

When sugars are ingested, the body produces insulin. This insulin enables circulation sugar to enter cells for utilisation as fuel. Consuming sugary meals may cause a quick spike in blood sugar that is followed by an insulin crash. Although an athlete may need a quick sugar boost during or just before a competition, consuming high-sugar meals in the days beforehand might cause an energy slump.

Foods with high sugar content include candy, doughnuts, certain granola bars, energy drinks, soda, cookies, cake, and other sweets. These goodies should be reserved for exceptional events on another day by an athlete.

Lastly, an athlete's digestive tract might be impacted by coffee and several supplements. On the day of the competition, an adolescent athlete should avoid using these items, particularly if they are new.

Are Eggs a Good Pre-Game Meal?

Teenagers may be reluctant to eat eggs before a game because of the legendary image in which Rocky Balboa drinks a raw egg shake during a strenuous training scenario. Rocky said it appeared to work?

A concentrated amount of high-quality protein, beneficial fats, and a dizzying assortment of vitamins and minerals can be found in eggs. In fact, they are the ideal supplement to a high-carb lunch or snack before a workout.

Yet, a few crucial rules turn eggs into a useful contribution rather than a performance inhibitor.
First off, athletes should never eat uncooked eggs. Eggs may absorb less protein and biotin if they are not cooked. More significantly, eating raw eggs puts you at risk for contracting a foodborne disease.

Second, meals before competitions should include more than simply eggs. Eggs include protein but no carbohydrate, a food that helps the body produce energy. The majority of the pre-game meal or snack should consist of carbohydrates, along with a modest quantity of protein, since they are the primary source of energy.

Lastly, because fat may upset the stomach, athletes should avoid using cooking techniques that add a lot of fat.

Best Tips for Fueling Pre-Workout

Best Tips for Fueling Pre-Workout